Happiness for
Sugar

Flip Smith

Happiness for Sugar
Copyright © 2020 by Flip Smith

All rights reserved. No part of this
publication may be reproduced, distributed,
or transmitted in any form or by any means,
including photocopying, recording, or
other electronic or mechanical methods,
without the prior written permission of
the author, except in the case of brief
quotations embodied in critical reviews
and certain other non-commercial
uses permitted by copyright law.

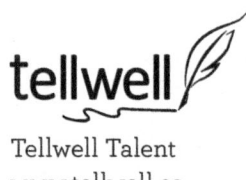

Tellwell Talent
www.tellwell.ca

ISBN
978-0-2288-2838-9 (Paperback)

The poetry book *Happiness for Sugar* is a book designed to make those feel like they can overcome any sadness that they have endured over their lifetime. It is there to guide people through their hard times and open the book when they need something to remind them that they can get through anything. It is there to show people the beauty of life, and the world around them. To show that whether it be in an airport or an elevator, people and interactions are important because it makes one realize how much love there is in this world. Most of all this book is designed to show someone that not a second of their life should be wasted because life is precious, and every single person brings a special light in the world.

Happiness for sugar

Sugar is like that bad habit that you can't beat,
You eat that candy,
Or add it to your tea,
You know this isn't good for you,
But you can't stop;
Sugar is a metaphor,
A metaphor for the bad,
Something you don't want to get rid of,
Because you love it too much,
But you know you're better off without it,
So, stop feeding your addiction of sugar,
Don't go back to it because once you overcome sugar,
You are free.

Elevators

Elevators are my favorite place,
Stepping into one,
While five others stand next to me,
Conversation has sparked,
A few jokes are said,
And as we stand there,
I find it refreshing knowing fate brought us all here in this moment,
And we begin to appreciate the power of human interaction,
The necessity of it,
as even just that conversation in the elevator,
may make someone's day,
their week,
or may save their life.

100 years from now

100 years from now,
No one will be left to remember you,
Your name, not known,
Your mark on the world, forgotten,
That smile of yours, no longer remembered,
And nothing you did will matter;
So, don't be afraid,
To live,
To die,
To be reckless,
To love unconditionally
Because 100 years from now,
No one will be left to remember you.

Music festivals

Drunker than ever,
Hearing the music connect with my body,
I dance,
Smiling as I gaze across the sea full of people,
And only in this moment,
Have I felt so connected with the world,
as I stand there,
While the music pulses through my body,
I realize, all of us listening,
We are all hear together,
As family.

Youth

As you grow,
You begin to understand the world,
The beauty of it,
And the horrors of it;
As you grow,
You have your whole life ahead of you,
The whole world in your hands;
So, don't make the mistake that so many of us do,
Don't waste a second of it,
And never do things halfway,
Pour your heart and soul into everything,
Don't be shy to do so,
Because the world needs your beauty,
Your kind heart,
And your energy.

Life

Life is a funny thing,
Too much time spent on the trivial things,
but instead we should be
Loving infinitively,
Acting spontaneously,
Sparking a fire in our heart,
And doing something that makes the adrenaline go wild in us,
because in the end,
life is a funny thing,
and it can be taken from us in a split second.

Brightest light

You are the brightest light,
Laughing unconditionally,
Blaring music,
Singing to it as loud as you could,
Your heart and soul was always 100%,
The kind to get a tattoo,
Travel across Europe,
Drop everything and move to a new town,
Compelling every kind of person to you,
The best kind,
Driving everyone to want to be as carefree,
Yet so full of life,
Thank you for teaching me how to live,
You are my brightest light.

Love and lose

You were here and then you weren't,
Wishing I could hold you one last time,
Hear that laugh,
Or see that smile,
Tell you how much beauty your heart held,
How much love you brought into the world,
You were the brightest light,
And now that light is gone,
And I will forever remember you,
Until we meet again.

Airports

Think of airports,
There is so much love,
In a world so damaged,
And hurting,
We fail to see the love that is all around us,
Whether it be that radiant smile as a loved one is reunited,
Or tears shed because one is leaving,
it is love,
So think of airports when you feel lost,
Because you will realize how much love there is,
In a world so damaged.

Two am thoughts

I loved all of you with every piece of my heart,
You lit a fire in me,
Making me feel more alive than I have ever felt,
You pushed me to be the best version of me I could ever be,
Every moment with you as spontaneous as ever,
But then you left,
And I'm here wondering,
if anyone could ever make me feel that way again.

You are in control

You are in control,
Of how you choose to live,
Who you let walk into your world,
And what you do with your life,
So choose your people,
Live only in pure happiness,
And do only the best you can,
Because anything less of this,
Is a life unfulfilled.

In the mirror

Often times you look in the mirror,
And I hear you point out all your imperfections,
Criticize yourself in cruel ways,
But the truth is,
The mirror is showing one of the most beautiful people of all,
and as you turn to me,
I know I am not the only one to think that,
There are no imperfections to be found,
But only you believe that to be wrong,
Because the one who sees themselves,
Is the one who is most critical.

The mind

The mind is the most powerful force of all with the control to alter how you think of yourself. So, my dear, don't let it tell you that you are anything short of perfect. The mind can be a tricky thing and one of the hardest to beat. So instead, wake up every day with the mindset to overcome any of the negatives because trust me when I say, there are only positives when it comes to you.

Pick yourself up

Life can be difficult,
And In the hardest of times,
You are the only one that can save you,
So, take care of yourself,
As after all the heartbreak and sadness,
Time will pass,
And eventually you will feel normal again,
Because you were there to remind you of how strong you are.

Choose colorful

In all the black and grey,
Choose colorful,
Wear that bright colored shirt,
Or socks,
Or beanie,
Because in a sea of grey and black,
Colorful may be exactly what someone needed to see.

Nights with friends

Don't take for granted those nights with friends,
Where you are up till 2am,
Laughing,
Crying,
Sneaking the wine into your room,
And dancing the night away,
Because those are the nights that you'll wish you could go back to,
When time has ticked away,
and all you are left with,
are memories to look back on.

Society

Society,
It tells us what our body size should be,
What we should wear,
And how we should act.
So much pressure put on all of us,
By the societal norms forced upon us,
And after a while,
We begin to care too much,
And everyone starts to wear and act the same,
But don't fall into this,
Because being you,
Is what is most important of all.

One day I wake up

One day I wake up,
All the pain is gone,
And I can breathe again,
My chest feels light,
My heart fills with joy,
So, I smile to myself,
And thank you for teaching me,
Just how strong I can be.

Some advice

Sometimes life hits hard. You could be having the best week, day, month, year of your life, and out of nowhere tragedy can instantly ruin that. Life takes its own course, and nothing can change one's own fate. Whether it be knowing what grief feels like, or depression, anxiety, or sexual assault. No one deserves to be put through it.

If you are reading this and have been through any of it, and are still here today, you are one of the strongest people to walk the earth. We do not know whether we are going to be here tomorrow, a week, or a year from now, so remind yourself in even the hardest of times, to get up and give 100% of you every single day.

Live everyday like it may be your last day as life is uncertain and it is important to make the most of it. Do something that you may be scared, shy, or hesitant to do every morning. Start your day off with a thrill and do something spontaneous. If life is so precious and can be taken in such an instant, don't waste your time.

Think of time as though it is the most delicate thing and only do with it the best that you can. Tell your friends and family that you love them. Do something for a stranger as you don't know what they have been through and the 100% you are giving of yourself everyday might just make their day. Life is short, life is precious, life is fun. So, don't waste a second on the unimportant.

Cities

Cities,
The most connected places,
Everywhere you go someone will be there,
Never alone,
But maybe the loneliest places,
Looking around,
A street of families,
Friends,
Not everyone may have this.

You

You,
My favorite kind of person,
Showed me what true love really is,
And here I am,
So glad that no one worked out before you,
Grateful for all the heart break,
Because without it,
There would be no you.

The next morning

In bed the next morning,
I lay there,
Wondering what happened the night before,
Foggy and unclear,
I realize someone had been in my room,
Uninvited,
And it wasn't you,
Despite knowing the pain that would come from this,
I knew I could get through this.

My favorite place

Coronas in hand,
Boats full of friends,
Music blaring,
and conversation with old friends,
pictures being taken,
it is the most therapeutic place,
as we all spend our day on the water,
together,
many things are appreciated,
and we realize the importance of home,
because home will always be there for us.

Mornings

Mornings,
The most exhilarating,
A whole day ahead,
And anything can happen,
It could be the best day of your life,
With new friends,
Or new ideas,
So, wake up every morning,
With only excitement,
And fall asleep at night,
Looking forward to the day that lies ahead.

The pain

Sometimes,
We think of pain,
The pain that everyone feels,
The tragedies that happen,
The struggles people go through,
And we ourselves feel this hurting,
Take on this burden,
And wish that we could take away this pain.

By chance

Isn't it crazy,
That by chance,
We end up where we are now,
Billions of people in the world,
Thousands of places to live,
Hundreds of ways our lives could have been different,
But we are here,
In this moment,
Purely by chance,
So, appreciate who is by your side,
because even if you walked into the wrong coffee shop,
you just might not have met them.

The world

If you feel lost,
Remember,
There is a whole world out there,
Pack up your stuff,
Move to a different town,
Get a new job,
Talk to new people,
Discover the world,
And when you have found your happiness,
And your people,
Call it home.

Forever

You excite me,
The way you are,
Goofy,
Funny,
And a little bit weird,
But your smile,
Your kiss,
And your quirky way of doing things,
Will forever have my heart.

Fire

You are like a fire,
Confined within a candle,
With the ability to be set free,
Overstep the boundaries,
And create a far bigger light within the world,
What's stopping you?

Breathe

The best feeling is when you breathe,
Really breathe for the first time in a while,
And it feels like nothing hurts anymore,
That breath is so refreshing,
Like a new start,
Because no longer is your mind filled with sadness,
Or your heart aching for happiness,
At last you are in the present,
That breath you just took,
Was the start of something new.

Dancing

Dance,
Whenever you can,
It is a sign of joy,
Dance your heart out,
Whether it be at parties,
or with your friends at 3am,
Because it's a way to say we are all connected,
And only in the purest and happiest of moments do we dance together.

Be different

In a world full of people,
Be different,
Embarrass yourself sometimes,
Be loud,
Be courageous,
Be confident,
And be passionate,
But most importantly,
Don't fit in,
Always be different.

Growth

The world holds so much hurting,
But you are like a flower within it,
Always growing,
Beautiful as ever.

Pay attention

Pay attention,
To those who are happy when you are,
Who check up on you,
And who mean it when they say they love you,
Because there is a difference between someone who means it,
And someone who says it.

Your worth

Know your worth,
You are amazing,
And anyone who treats you as less than this,
Is someone who fails to see how beautiful your heart is.

Broken

After a while,
I realized how I should be treated,
Your actions shattering me,
Your words cutting deep,
Knowing I deserved better,
I could no longer stay.

Signs

I saw all the signs,
But I chose to ignore them,
Because you were like a drug,
And I was addicted.

Your path

Where you are now,
May not be where you are in 2 years,
Life takes its own course,
And what is meant to happen,
Will happen,
So, stress less,
And let life take you where it needs to.

Technology

In a place with so much technology,
We fail to remember that human interaction is the most powerful of all,
So please put your phone down,
Talk to someone new,
Read a book,
Go outside and appreciate the world around you.

Passion

Find what you love,
And once you do,
Give it your all,
Be as passionate as you can,
And make sure to express this passion,
By doing this,
It'll bring joy to the people around you,
As seeing your passion,
And your heart so full,
Will light up someone's world.

www.ingramcontent.com/pod-product-compliance
Lightning Source LLC
LaVergne TN
LVHW042004060526
838200LV00041B/1869